# Table of Contents

The Role of Antibiotics in Treating Rosacea Symptoms: A Comprehensive Review

# 5.2. Exploring the Potential of Probiotics in Rosacea Management

# The Efficacy of Antibiotics in Treating Rosacea

# 1. Introduction to Rosacea

The American Academy of Dermatology has established the following diagnostic criteria: flushing, redness, pimples, and visible blood vessels. Eye signs include dry eyes, burning or stinging, ropy discharge, swelling, and other eye symptoms. Rosacea is a chronic, inflammatory, non-contagious, swelling condition that affects the skin of the face. It typically starts as redness in the cheeks and nose that comes and goes. Over time, the redness becomes ruddier and more persistent, and visible blood vessels may appear. Left untreated, pimples and bumps may develop, or, in part, the nose may grow swollen from excess tissue. The keys to avoiding rosacea discomfort include avoiding skin products that irritate the skin or cause flushing, medications, red wine, and extreme weather.

Rosacea is a common and chronic skin condition of the face that is characterized by redness, bumps, pimples, and visible blood vessels. It can affect anybody, but it is most commonly seen in individuals in their 30s. Men are more likely to suffer from rosacea. Rosacea is not contagious, but it is misunderstood and can be an emotional problem because the redness of the skin makes people feel embarrassed and uncomfortable. An estimated 16 million Americans suffer from rosacea, and around 415 million globally. Although it is a common condition, many people do not know much about it. More than 90% of individuals do not know what rosacea is, what it appears to be, or how it is treated, according to the National Rosacea Society.

## 1.1. Definition and Symptoms

The redness, intense flushing, inflammation, and visible blood vessel formations associated with rosacea-like conditions could be treated with procedures like lasers and intense pulsed light therapy. In mild to moderate cases, antibiotics such as oral doxycycline have been found to reduce the severity of rosacea. However, a sub-antimicrobial dose of various tetracyclines has been applied to patients for years to minimize and control rosacea-like signs and symptoms. Bringing the subject back to rosacea, the worst outcome over time, according to experts, might be the appearance of ocular symptoms. It has been estimated that 60% of all rosacea sufferers will go on to contract ocular rosacea. Even individuals who have only mild rosacea on their facial skin may eventually go on to develop significant eye disease, and we may even see this in teenagers.

Rosacea is a common chronic dermatological disorder that predominantly occurs on the central area of the face. The pathogenesis of this skin condition has been researched quite extensively, but the cause is still unknown. However, various triggering factors have been identified including exposure to the sun, heat, cold, wind, and stress. People of all origins, skin types, and colors can develop rosacea. The symptoms often begin with frequent flushing and gradually develop into more persistent redness and visible blood vessels on the face. Left untreated, pimples and bumps often develop, and in severe cases, the nose may grow swollen and bumpy from excess tissue.

## 1.2. Prevalence and Impact

It can affect the mental and functional elements of public life. Previous queries revealed that a substantive proportion of people had discontinued functioning due to the disorder. The social life of nearly two-thirds of the victims was impacted. Patients also seek support for the psychological pressure they are under. In a previous survey, the victims were found to break out of functioning due to rosacea changes. Loss of work results from disruption of day-long morale, depression, and confidence in oneself. Patients were aware of their issues which were under-treated and had a lot of interest in others, and rosacea was recognized as a main reason for lack of self-reliance and self-confidence. All of the above causes make rosacea an engaging issue in need of treatment and research. The found effect of rosacea disorder on individuals' lives justifies antibiotic therapy for vascular rosacea, as modern therapeutic solutions frequently will.

Although rosacea is very prevalent among the general public, the true incidence in the Western world and in Japan is unknown, according to a published article. Rosacea is an inflammatory, chronic condition that may have marked practical and emotional implications for those suffering from it. Rosacea is frequently covered, and its pulmonary effects are very remarkable. Papulopustular and pyoinflammatory rosacea coincide with the frequency of adverse impact on quality of life. Ocular changes and seborrhea concurrent with rhinophyma were reported to have additionally affected the outcome.

## 2. Antibiotics as Treatment for Rosacea

In order to help you understand the efficacy of antibiotics in treating rosacea, let's start by explaining their mechanisms of action. Tetracyclines, macrolides, and metronidazole are the antibiotics traditionally used to tackle rosacea, acting not only as antibacterial but also anti-inflammatory properties. Tetracyclines reduce inflammation through a number of pathways. As intracellular enzymes that degrade chemical mediators inducing inflammation are modified, the additional presence of tetracycline prevents this degradation and reduces the incidence and intensity of inflammation, which leads to visible symptoms such as papules. They also inhibit the migration of neutrophils and prevent the release of pro-inflammatory enzymes and metabolites. Macrolides, through their action on protein synthesis, inhibit the release of proteins that are involved with cell signaling and subsequent degradation of molecules inducing inflammation. Lastly, metronidazole may inhibit the growth of certain bacteria responsible for initiating the inflammation, which manifests as pustules, papules, flushing, and dilation of the blood vessels. It is actively being diluted in the body and may also reduce the incidence and severity of some of the visible symptoms.

Having discussed what rosacea is and its different types, the next question worth discussing is: can rosacea be cured with antibiotics? The simple answer to this question is yes, it can. It is important to remember, though, that antibiotics aren't a cure for rosacea. However, they are anti-inflammatory and can be an effective treatment to manage the condition and symptoms.

## 2.1. Mechanisms of Action

Another mechanism of action of antibiotics is through anti-inflammatory action; by being absorbed into the human body, the antibiotic provides anti-inflammatory effects against the systemic and local inflammation, while also continuing to exhibit anti-inflammatory effects directly against the local vascular microbiome. The fourth mechanism (and often omitted consideration) is the anti-fibrotic and anti-papule formation action of antibiotics: through the administration of sub-antimicrobial doses of a sub-antimicrobial antibiotic plated against rosacea-associated microorganisms (SARAMEC). By coming to an understanding of the mechanisms of action, antibiotics (and the health professionals who opt to include antibiotics as part of the treatment regimen) appear as consonant coadjutors in a basic regimen that attacks rosacea particularly where it needs to be treated.

The most broadly well-known mechanism of action (MOA) for antibiotics in the treatment of rosacea is the antibiotic's ability to attack the microorganism and usually decrease the density of inflammatory-inducing Demodex mites. The second MOA is the direct antimicrobial effect the antibiotic exerts against the vascular microbiome in the dermis of the facial skin. Both of these MOAs are temporary in their effects if the antibiotic therapy is stopped and are currently seen as mechanisms of management: the antibiotics provide long-term control over symptoms but not a cure.

## 2.2. Types of Antibiotics Used

Two of the most commonly used classes of antibiotics are macrolides and tetracyclines. Erythromycin base and its stearate and ethylsuccinate esters, like lymphostasis, is a macrolide that can be taken systemically or used topically in a 2% concentration. Because they have similar action to macrolides, lincomycin and clindamycin can also be used to treat rosacea. The oral forms of these antibiotics are only available. However, the patient will have more chance of developing pseudomembranous colitis and diarrhea if taking cleocin orally than if erythromycin is taken, due to clindamycin's negative side effects which are not present in erythromycin. Clarithromycin, a macrolide similar to erythromycin that has an expanded spectrum of action, is only available orally and has been linked to an increase in eosinophil infiltrates when taken at 500 mg twice per day. Rosacea is generally treated with antibiotics such as tetracycline and minocycline, which work by killing papuetary acne, reducing inflammation, and reducing pain. However, it has been shown that various bacteria associated with rosacea are resistant to antibiotics.

Once bacterium has been linked to the pathogenesis of rosacea, there have been many investigations into the efficacy of antibiotic use for this skin disease. Various types of antibiotics have been studied for their applications. Both oral and topical types have been employed, and although not all antibiotics have shown significant results, there are many promising drugs. This section will overview the types of antibiotics that are often used for these diseases, including macrolides and tetracyclines, cephalosporins, and fluoroquinolones.

# 3. Clinical Studies and Evidence

Erythromycin, isotretinoin, tetracyclines, and doxycycline are potential groundbreaking treatments for extensive papulopustular and phymatous rosacea. As part of antimicrobial use, we also documented the efficacy of the 50-year-old compound metronidazole in caring for remission of and effectively preventing rosacea relapse. Owing to the potential definitive side effects of isotretinoin such as cheilitis, nasal dryness, skin pruritus, xerosis, dry throat, and disease, this care is often treated with other drugs. Furthermore, isotretinoin is considered "an exceptional second-line treatment" for potential adult women instances who are not planned to conceive but who are unable to take an effective drug, considering multiple aspects.

For about 5 decades, several clinical studies have sought to determine the efficacy, safety, and potential mechanisms addressing the role of local and systemic antibiotics in the care of different rosacea phenotypes. The evidence suggests that both oral and topical antibiotics are used for all rosacea phenotypes, though this is off-label for erythematotelangiectatic rosacea. The trials indicate that the use of antibiotics present in two meta-analyses is clearly significant but small for papulopustular/vascular rosacea. Antimicrobial agents are widely used in rosacea care and show significant efficacy, but their use is limited to no more than 4-8 months since their recurrence is unpredictable. However, many studies have strongly suggested a potential financial and ecological risk of these solutions. Other possible mechanisms are of particular relevance in subgroups. Micronutrients and antioxidants are other good candidates to act as adjuncts/focused contraceptives and are considered well by patients.

## 3.1. Overview of Key Studies

The authors concluded that the antibiotic was effective in reducing the inflammatory rosacea over the short-term. There is some evidence that azithromycin exhibits superior efficiency over longer treatment duration. Finally, the systemic antibiotic appears to be effective for redness associated with disease. Possible differences in efficacy between systemic and low-dose doxycycline are not clear. The authors suggested that the low quality of evidence and small sample size of the studies included limit the generalizability of their conclusions. Hence, this review does not clarify the position of the antibiotics and the preferred dose for rosacea based on high-quality evidence. Given the concerns regarding chronic antibiotics, this suggests that the need for chronic, potentially lifetime antibiotics needs to be carefully balanced against the low quality of the evidence.

In contrast, no difference was found between low-dose doxycycline and azithromycin in any of the time period groups. Finally, Liu et al. (2020) found that low-dose doxycycline was as effective as ivermectin 1% cream for reducing papulopustular rosacea over 16 weeks; reduction in erythema was also similar between the two groups. An additional study by the same author found that low-dose doxycycline did not have less efficacy in reducing erythema when compared with azithromycin 250 mg/day, despite the lower incidence of bacterial resistance.

According to Jansen et al. (2003), doxycycline 100 mg is statistically and clinically superior to minocycline, oxytetracycline, and placebo in treating inflammatory rosacea. However, this conclusion is based on several limitations, including lack of blinding, inadequate sample size, and selection bias. Moore et al. (2006) showed that doxycycline 40 mg and 20 mg are clinically and statistically superior to placebo in treating inflammatory rosacea. Besides, shortages of other available oral antibiotics were noted. Pancar et al. (2017) compared the efficiency of low-dose doxycycline (40 mg/day), systemic metronidazole, and oral azithromycin. Both doxycycline and metronidazole caused a reduction in the severity of the disease over 28 days, and the difference in efficacy between these two agents was not significant. Oral azithromycin was shown to have significant clinical and statistical efficacy in the treatment of inflammatory rosacea. Two months after treatment, azithromycin was found to have significantly superior effectiveness compared to the other two common agents.

This review aimed to determine the place of antibiotics in managing rosacea by conducting a narrative review of relevant data. The authors examined the efficacy of topical and systemic antibiotic treatment and preferred antibiotics used at doxycycline, tetracycline, minocycline, and lymecycline doses. Key study findings included the following.

3.1. Overview of key studies

# Antibiotics analysis for the management of rosacea: Deconstructing the evidence

## 3.2. Effectiveness and Safety

2. Most of the cosmetics and sunscreens were found to be helpful in reducing both the intense background erythema and flushing in general and the transient flushing after stimuli such as exposure to indirect heat or exercise. The serious complications by leaving papulopustules without treatment to avoid the promoters of the disease have not been studied.

1. There are individuals affected with pimples, pustules, and erythema that did not respond to antibiotic therapy and were found to have no Demodex follicular nor any other cause in their skin scraping or in a biopsy taken from the most erythematous area. In those individuals, rosacea seemed to result from inappropriate development and functioning of the immune system. Phototherapy, lasers, and IPL were found to be most helpful. At present, the only oral or topical products well studied for the long-term treatment of papulopustules are the anti-parasitic agents metronidazole and ivermectin. Antibiotics such as azithromycin and modulators such as spironolactone may have a similar effect in papulopustules but have hardly been studied yet.

3.2. Effectiveness of Antibiotics in Rosacea

The evidence regarding the efficacy, safety, and potential for resistance to antibiotics has been key in the management of rosacea.

# 4. Combination Therapies

# 4.1. Antibiotics with Topical Treatments

# 4.2. Antibiotics with Oral Medications

# 5. Antibiotic Resistance in Rosacea Treatment

Are oral antibiotics no longer an acceptable treatment in rosacea? While this is a widely held viewpoint in dermatology, this notion may need revision, especially in the context of highly structured, short-term regimens for the conversion of subtype 2 erythematotelangiectatic rosacea to predominantly 1:1: erythematotelangiectatic/papulopustular/phymatous rosacea prior to utilizing longer-term topicals. Once-daily doxycycline 40 mg as monotherapy given continuously for 6 months is of benefit in the treatment of moderate-to-severe papulopustular rosacea (including its four subtypes, 1:1, 0:1, 1:0:1, and 1:1:1) in healthy adults, with an NNT of 7 (6-9) for at least 'marked improvement' (more than 70% reduction from baseline in lesions, erythema, or both combined). Sub-optimal doses of daily doxycycline below 40 mg are generally ineffective. Therefore, while the efficacy of doxycycline at a dose of 40 mg/day has not been directly compared with a higher dose of this doxycycline formulation or any standard doxycycline dose (i.e., below 40 mg) to date, a non-systematic review of the literature found that the available data on systemic deworming, wound care, and antimicrobial therapy supported the use of this dose for prolonged periods. A 60 mg daily dose of doxycycline was not superior to a 40 mg daily dose in the treatment of severe facial acne vulgaris in two short-term (3- and 4-month) randomized controlled trials.

Antibiotic resistance in the management of a chronic, recurrent condition There is substantial concern regarding the rise of antibiotic resistance as a consequence of long-term antibiotic use for the treatment of chronic and recurrent conditions, with potential consequences for public health. Rosacea is a chronic and recurrent disease; while symptoms may be diminished with treatment, rosacea is unlikely to be cured. As such, the implications of using oral antimicrobials long term in rosacea are of particular interest.

# 6. Future Directions and Research Opportunities

Emerging Therapies. Almost all emerging therapies for rosacea are directed towards the pathogenesis of the disease. A therapeutic development pipeline has been identified for rosacea that includes topical brimonidine, systemic anti-inflammatory medications, and immunomodulatory agents (including biologics). Since we have identified well-studied first- and second-line systemic anti-inflammatory medications for rosacea—the tetracyclines in particular—research opportunities will continue to exist for newer antibiotics and anti-inflammatory medications. Given that aberrant immune responses are involved in the pathogenesis of rosacea, the development of new immunomodulatory agents for rosacea is likely to become an important research area in the future. In addition, personalized approaches to therapy are under clinical investigation for many diseases and are likely to be more rigorously studied in the treatment of rosacea as we garner better understanding of its pathogenesis and identify endotypes. The ultimate goals of these newer therapies or personalized approaches would be to create fewer adverse effects, elicit quicker onset of action, have easier methods of administration, and, of course, increased long-term efficacy against the development or progression of rosacea.

In conclusion, short-term application of tetracyclines will produce benefits. The use of non-antibiotics has also been effective in recent studies. Interestingly, only synthetic tetracyclines with low antibiotic potency are effective against rosacea, and the efficacy of doxycycline less than 40mg cannot be accurately evaluated due to insufficient evidence. Likewise, due to insufficient evidence, the new slow-release doxycycline is used for the treatment of ocular rosacea and the other proposed combination therapy. However, these inactive tetracyclines suggest a possible relation between the anti-inflammatory activity of crystalline tetracyclines and the pathogenesis of rosacea, especially since early diagnosis has shown the absence of focal or circumscribed infections, and newer therapeutic concepts have proposed the role of increased innate immunity and inflammation in this disease. Personalized treatment appears to be the main research area for the development of new therapies, including personalized selection of systemic treatments for certain rosaceas and localization of pregnant women.

This review provided a comprehensive overview of the efficacy of antibiotics in the management of rosacea. More well-constructed and rigorous studies are needed in the future to help guide clinical treatment. The conclusion of this review is intended to provide a reference for future studies and new therapies for the treatment of rosacea.

## 6.1. Emerging Therapies

Oral medication Topical medication Other therapeutic modalities Oral medication evaluated and included, we present new drugs, off-label uses, and combined treatments effective in a small number of studies by the American Academy of Dermatology. Subantimicrobial-dose doxycycline (modified-release doxycycline) has a favorable effect in the subset of patients with a severe inflammatory component that warrants the use of an oral drug, including rosacea patients with proven papules and pustules; the latter is particularly indicated when pregnancy is not excluded. In the same context, small studies with azithromycin have been conducted evaluating the safety and efficacy of a low dose (400 mg for three days every week for three weeks). Antibiotics may have been curative not only by virtue of their ability to suppress bacteria but also through their effect of anti-inflammation, an idea that could also have a wider application for other common inflammatory skin disorders. If the latter suggestion is confirmed, they will have provided an answer to the dilemmas raised by rosacea therapy. Similarly, an anti-inflammatory action has been described in the new immunosuppressive drugs, which decrease inflammatory mediators, cytokines, and T-cell proliferation, namely PDE-4 inhibitors and JAK-1-2 inhibitors, holding promise for the future.

Over the past decades, a number of new dermatologic treatment modalities have been developed, accelerating the progress of antibiotic resistance. The concept of current management uses emerging therapies as active, anti-inflammatory medications acting to control our treatment goals. This will likely result in the decay of the pathogenic targets, with researchers effectively responsible for the disease in patients, instead of achieving complete bacterial suppression during the whole therapy, over and above being effective antibiotics. The novel approach that new therapeutic modalities offer represents a futuristic transition in effective rosacea treatment management from the antibiotic-based therapy of the past to antibiotic-sparing management in clinical years to come. If the role of non-antibiotic (non-antimicrobial) therapies is demonstrated, it will have resolved a long-standing worry of the struggling antibiotic industry, which has so far hamstrung the progress that has been made in exploring non-antibiotics for many years in rosacea.

## 6.2. Personalized Medicine Approaches

Rosacea is a diversifiable disorder that can present with combinations, shades, and sequences of the four major clinical subtypes of rosacea. Rosacea can be influenced by several trigger factors at once or can be dependent on multiple trigger factors. Rosacea therapy should be subtyped from classification features to the individual patient. As the therapeutic approach to rosacea, including sebopsoriasis, is chosen based on the principles and methods of personalized medicine, this approach is shaped for the patient's non-disease characteristics—pH and skin surface position pH, sebum position and amount, keratinography, etiopathogenesis, etc., and for non-rosacea-trigger and rosacea-trigger results. Antibiotics used as monotherapy efficacy or for rosacea benefits are established in clinical trials.

Personalized medicine approaches might help find an optimized way to use antibiotics for rosacea treatment, aiming to prevent antibiotic abuse and the basic principles of treating severe and emerging rosacea cases on an individual healthcare plan for all rosacea classifications. Rosacea is a chronic, relapsing dermatological condition. The efficacy and role of antibiotics for rosacea remain unquestionable, but perhaps combining antibiotics with other rosacea treatments and individually prolonging the discontinuous regime or maintaining anti-rosacea responding and drug resistance can be a more successful therapeutic approach against rosacea according to the personalized medicine concept.

# The Role of Antibiotics in Treating Rosacea Symptoms: A Comprehensive Review

# 1. Introduction to Rosacea and Antibiotics

Rosacea is an inflammatory skin disorder with multiple factors that occur only on the human face. The primary symptoms of the disease are flushing, persistent central facial erythema, papules, and pustules. Less common ocular symptoms, such as burning or stinging, gritty or sandy feeling, itching, photophobia, or vision disturbances, can also be observed and are considered specific for rosacea. Once considered to be pathognomonic, the presence of demodex folliculorum is now widely reported but not unequivocally confirmed. The microbiota change (also known as dysbiosis) is now to the detriment of protective attributes. Neither causal relationships nor the sequence of rosacea between innate and adaptive immunity, nor genetic susceptibility, is currently understood.

Rosacea, a chronic relapsing inflammatory skin disease, affects millions of people in the world. Antibiotics have long been used to manage inflammatory papulopustular and erythematotelangiectatic rosacea. The main drugs used to reduce inflammation and prevent relapses have recently included new drugs. They can be used alone or in sequential multitreatment, and they include doxycycline, minocycline, azithromycin, trimethoprimsulfamethoxazole, topical ivermectin, and topical metronidazole. Currently, patients are seeking alternative therapies to avoid antibiotic use due to concerns over the potential risks associated with long-term use, including drug resistance and changes to microbiota. This article aims to provide an up-to-date overview of the role and potential advantages of antibiotics in the treatment of rosacea symptoms. Furthermore, considering the descriptive and critical characteristics, the paper could also be useful for those planning to conduct systematic reviews. If future research is planned, it may be useful to define the structured search string and critical information on toxicological aspects.

## 1.1. Understanding Rosacea: Causes, Symptoms, and Triggers

The four distinct primary symptoms of rosacea vary in descriptiveness and possess different levels of severity. A relatively akin erythematotelangiectatic rosacea can result from the areas of visible dwelling in some patients. As a result, facial redness (blushing) typically goes together with this type of rosacea. Patients who suffer from rosacea are known to complain of temporary or permanent facial redness. The cheeks, nostrils, or the entire face can be swarmed by this redness. In the proposed studies, 76 percent of rosacea cohort research members showed signs of facial swelling due to redness.

Rosacea is a common skin condition primarily observed in adults that is characterized by excessive redness, visible blood vessels, pimples, and red bumps on the skin in the face. The nose, cheeks, and chin, as well as the forehead and scalp, have been documented as areas typically affected by rosacea, and the chest, ears, and neck can also experience these symptoms. The condition does not have a known cause and is typically observed more frequently in women, although when observed in men, the symptoms appear to be more severe. A proposed but ultimately inconclusive cause of rosacea is the overgrowth of small organisms in the patient's skin. One distinct category—Demodex folliculorum mites—has been the specific target of a particular hypothesis over the past decade, as two similar studies identified it as a more dominant microorganism in rosacea patients compared to those without rosacea. Parasite sensitivity, unrelated studies have found, can also make the skin very itchy and result in additional red rashes that can create rough, dry, and scaly skin infiltrations on the face. Additionally, rosacea symptoms can progress in severity and may ultimately cause fibrous or granulomatous disorders (a substantial growth in sebaceous glands), and rosacea may also cause the nose to appear swollen.

## 1.2. Mechanisms of Action of Antibiotics in Treating Rosacea

In patients with rosacea, the number of effective mites in the skin and eyes decreased after oral antibiotics, and the number of patients with erythromelalgia in the eyes decreased. During the 4 to 8 weeks, papules on the skin and spiders began to subside, and the skin was smooth and the skin elasticity improved. In the chronic stage of recalcitrant rosacea, even if the number of mites reaches or increases to a large extent, the patient's skin itching, erythema, and swelling subside. There are also reports of some patients who use external antibiotics for a few months, and nasal congestion and skin pimples are still significantly reduced and improved. The reduction of radionuclide concentration or the local area marker in rosacea patients reveals that demodex skin symptoms are significantly improved. These indicate that the antibacterial effect of demodex is the main mechanism by which demodex improves skin symptoms in patients with facial erythema acne. Some patients have mild to moderate keratosis skin diseases. The doctor used oral antibiotics to reduce facial erythema acne and found that the damage to the skin demons had also improved. In view of the above, demodex's improvement in the symptoms of rosacea is largely due to the removal of bacteria or other substances on the skin or in the inflammation of the hair follicles. Administering oral antibacterial drugs can also inhibit the growth of bacteria in hair follicles that use topically applied external antibiotics. More research should be done in the future to understand the mechanism by which antibiotic treatment for demodex removes skin inflammation.

Rosacea shows keratitis, mainly due to chronic inflammation of the face and sebaceous glands. The clinical phenomena are small pimples on the face, congestion on the forehead, a large number of worm-like small arteries on the nose and cheeks, and superficial papillary swelling. Edema, itching, hot and tingling sensation in the eye area, some patients may even develop seborrheic dermatitis or dry dermatitis. The treatments of rosacea include topical medications, oral drugs, or phototherapy. Rosacea's facial skin can be used to fight demodex with antibiotics. The mechanism may be to inhibit the mite bacillus around the hair follicle and hair worm, and reduce the mites and other bacteria in the hair follicles and sebaceous glands, reduce local inflammation, stabilize keratin cell proliferation and differentiation, and promote hair follicle epithelium basal synthesis of keratin fibers.

## 2. Commonly Used Antibiotics for Rosacea Treatment

2. Commonly Used Antibiotics for Rosacea Treatment. Rosacea treatment consists of a wide range of drugs for different patient profiles, mainly dedicated to topical therapy and adjuvant care using oral therapies in limited cases. In recent years, with increasing antibiotic resistance level, the use of oral antibiotics has slightly decreased. In the case of subtype 2 and 4, the evidence of improvement is still higher with pharmacological therapy, especially with oral antibiotics, associated with a wide variety of anti-inflammatory agents. Tetracyclines (doxycycline, tetracycline, lymecycline, and minocycline) are the gold standard and the most used oral antibiotics in normal clinical practice. Used in their modified release, they have an absorbable correlation. Tetracyclines not only have antibacterial activities but also have a wide variety of immune-modulating effects, including the suppression of matrix metalloproteinase and chemotactic factors. They can also reduce reactive nitrogen and oxygen species production by acting as scavengers and preventing some cells destruction. The anti-inflammatory dose must only be half the dose used for antimicrobial activity. One possible explanation originally suggests that tetracycline could reduce the production of matrix metalloproteinase by neutrophils at low dosages. Because of their widespread use and the potential for other conditions such as dental/orthopedics and reproductive health, within the

first stage of the inflammatory pathway, the importance of tetracyclines is undoubtable. At higher dosages, all tetracyclines can be bactericidal, but at sub-antimicrobial doses, they can act as a bacteriostatic drug. The advantages of doxycycline are the shorter half-life and better consumer tolerance compared to other tetracyclines. Although pustules have been reported to be more affected, they all have the same effect on the reduction of inflammatory lesions. A possible adverse effect of tetracycline mentioned is the potential for photosensitivity. Macrolides, erythromycin, and clarithromycin are considered acceptable alternatives, but the guidelines do not recommend their use due to the high level of resistance and low evidence of beneficial response compared to tetracyclines. The minimum erythromycin inhibitory concentration (MIEC) for Propionibacterium acnes and Staphylococcus aureus have been suspiciously reported. Owing to an absence of investment in their conception, including large-scale trials of antibiotics, drugs have been little exploited for the prevention of antibiotic-resistant staining or re-colonization in normal flora.

Up until the present date, antibiotics undoubtedly play a significant role in reducing inflammatory lesions and relieving other symptoms in rosacea patients. Due to different outcomes in practice and current discrepancy between guidelines, it is challenging to understand the exact position of antibiotic therapy in the rosacea treatment pathway. This paper provides literature-based knowledge about the role of systemic antibiotics including tetracyclines and alternatives such as macrolides, and provides an overview that also addresses topical inhibitors and current molecules in development.

## 2.1. Tetracyclines: Doxycycline and Minocycline

Doxycycline, which is considered a long-acting drug in comparison to other tetracyclines with a longer half-life of about 18-22 hours, also functions as an immune modulator and can inhibit the proliferation of human T-lymphocytes. Doxycycline prevents metalloproteinase (especially that of matrix-degrading enzyme) by chelating metal ions including zinc and calcium. Moreover, it also exhibits potent inhibition of neutrophil chemotaxis and reactive oxygen species (ROS). MC is devoid of lipid side chains; therefore, unlike doxycycline, it does not bind to tissues, but can easily diffuse across biological membranes enhancing intracellular concentration. It also acts by inhibiting protein synthesis by binding to the 30S ribosomal subunit in the cells and it functions as a kinase inhibitor or apoptosis inhibitor. However, prolonged use of tetracyclines alters the subcellular localization of the NF-κB and leads to inhibition of its activity and translocation to the nucleus of the cells. Hence, these tetracyclines are suggested to be known as non-specific immunomodulators.

Both doxycycline (DC) and minocycline (MC) have the capability of providing good therapeutic benefits in the treatment of rosacea since they carry anti-inflammatory, antiangiogenic, antioxidative, anti-apoptotic, and free-radical scavenging effects in the therapy of dermatological disorders. However, the use of MC or doxycycline may pose risks and challenges during skin therapy, as they can cause increased photosensitivity and several side effects including deposition of pigmentation.

## 2.2. Macrolides: Erythromycin and Azithromycin

Azithromycin is a bacteriostatic antibiotic of the macrolide family, with a long half-life that allows conquests in a few days. Currently, the effects of treatment with systemic azithromycin have been proven in the literature through numerous studies. Azithromycin improved from the sixth therapy day associated with a more increases on cutaneous population of Lactobacillus. Azithromycin used as alternative treatment regimens improved the QoL. Azithromycin showed a similar efficacy to doxycycline (100 mg once a day) and equally prevented relapses once the antibiotic therapy was suspended. The effectiveness of azithromycin therapy in the long term was also shown after the suspension of the antibiotic treatment: the 8-week relapse rate was 41% in the azithromycin group and 36% in the topical azelaic acid group.

Erythromycin is an antibiotic that has been reported to display an anti-inflammatory action in addition to its bacteriostatic effect. As compared with other antibiotics of the macrolide family, erythromycin has a lower tissue penetration, which makes it less interesting for the treatment of systemic infections. Topical erythromycin 2% gel (Erygel) was the first FDA-approved product in 1989 for the treatment of papulopustular rosacea. The efficacy of erythromycin topical product was demonstrated in two 11-week, weekly pare review of cleanser, an in topical metronidazole order to or placebo-controlled studies. A phase 3 clinical trial showed that patients using azelaic acid 15% twice daily experienced a 50% reduction on the

Investigator Global Assessment (IGA) of rosacea in as soon as 4 weeks. In addition, AzA 15%, at 15% also improves the inflammatory pain and burning associated with rosacea.

## 2.3. Topical Antibiotics: Metronidazole and Clindamycin

In endemic rosacea, topical agents are recommended alone or in combination with systemic drugs (doxycycline/oracea, tetracycline, isotretinoin, metronidazole) for papules and pustules. This mix can enhance the benefits of topical treatments acting on the inflammatory process (TNFα and IFNγ inhibition). Topical treatments are frequently used in a split-face style, comparing the effective skin half sides to the control sides to illustrate two therapies' potential differences.

Treatment selections are directed towards the symptoms, magnitude, etiology, and disease's duration. While relying on several classification methods, they involve: ingredient or form of medication, action target on the pathological mechanism, location of action, local or systemic impact, or class of drug. The agreed-upon classification standards for rosacea treatment involve both disease pathophysiology and response to treatment. This suggests that it is challenging to design and standardize particular protocols.

The significance of topical antibiotics: Topical antibiotics can be used to treat rosacea. The application of standard doses to punctually cover the lesion improves the complete and moderate relief of the disease. This is the conclusion of a systematic review and meta-analysis published by Cochrane in 2007. There are reported transdermal equivalent doses to homemade preparations: a 1% concentration of metronidazole or clindamycin gel or cream in adults and children with a mean age of 17 and 42.6 years reduces facial erythema and inflammatory lesions. The evidence is still limited, but these antibiotics are suitable as a first-line treatment. There are no important adverse events recorded for either children or adults. Topical antibiotics can be purchased by the patient.

Topical antibiotics - such as metronidazole and clindamycin 1% - are first-line treatments prescribed by the National Institute for Health and Care Excellence (NICE) and the Global Rosacea Consensus (GRAC) group guidelines. They can be safely used in adults and children with a mean age of 17 (5 to 45 years) and 42.6 years (34.3 to 55.5 years), respectively. These antibiotics inhibit or kill the bacteria responsible for developing the disease, thus improving the cutaneous side effects in most patients.

## 3. Efficacy and Safety of Antibiotics in Rosacea Treatment

Rosacea is a chronic inflammatory condition that primarily affects the face and blood vessels, constituting an important pathology in the practice of dermatology and aesthetic medicine. A wide range of therapeutic strategies based on clinical signs and symptoms is used for rosacea treatment, including general oral and/or topical medication and procedures like light/laser systems, etc. Probably due to the high prevalence of some bacterial subtypes in these patients, antibiotic treatments have also been found to be effective in clinical practice. Given the side effects and contraindications of classic systemic antibiotics (particularly tetracyclines and macrolides), there is a great need to find drugs from molecules and new technologies (e.g., peptides, liposomes, use of bacteria in the form of microorganisms, photodynamic therapy) that reduce systemic toxicity and enzymes to develop antimicrobial resistance (AMR) in patients with rosacea.

Rosacea is a common chronic skin disease for which antibiotics are often prescribed. Although the European and Russian professional leagues of dermatology recommend the use of antibiotics and the American Academy for Dermatology specifies them as a suggested treatment, there is no doubt that a critical approach to the efficacy-safety ratio and the pertinence of choosing such treatment in rosacea therapy is mandatory. We performed a comprehensive review of cohort studies, case control studies, randomized controlled trials, extensive reviews of the literature as well as case reports, clinical trials, and in vitro and in vivo tests in healthy patients, patients with rosacea, or animal models with rosacea that were performed to establish the efficacy and safety of antibiotic treatment for the symptoms of the disease. Although light and laser-based treatments are now firmly indicated in the management of rosacea, the evidence-based evaluation of the antibiotics mostly used in rosacea patients is of pivotal importance for therapeutic decisions.

## 3.1. Clinical Studies and Evidence-Based Findings

To emphasize, 20 mg/day doxycycline in Oraycea™ is not consistently effective in treating rosacea by providing both antibacterial and anti-inflammatory action, although the results are superior to those of placebo based on labeling and early clinical trials. In general, promoting the anti-inflammatory effectiveness of doxycycline while minimizing adverse events is likely to be superior to emphasizing anti-inflammatory benefits.

Over the years, rosacea has been effectively treated with various dosages of immediate-release oral doxycycline and its modified-release forms, such as 40 mg Dox, 30 mg Dox, and 1 mg doxycycline 30 mg. Rosacea experts agree that there is no single best dose of doxycycline for rosacea management. Doxycycline is usually prescribed in treatment doses not less than 40 mg/day for multiple months until the anatomic lesions of rosacea have gone. It is advisable to titrate the dose to avoid excessive adverse events in older individuals with more comorbidities. For antibacterial activity, the dose is generally 40 mg/day. For anti-inflammatory doses, the recommendation is 30 mg/day.

In a double-blind, randomized, controlled study lasting 4 weeks, Prosad™ cream (0.05% nimodipine and 2.5% metronidazole) was found to be effective in reducing inflammatory lesions, improving erythema, and quality of life in 68 adults with moderate-to-severe papulopustular rosacea who were divided into two equal groups and treated with vehicle combined with 0.75% metronidazole cream and 0.05% nimodipine (treatment group) or saline cream and 0.75% metronidazole cream.

The treatment of rosacea can be achieved by addressing each of the pathophysiologic mechanisms of the disease, such as demodex mites, dysregulation of innate and adaptive immunity, changes in the inflammatory cytokines of the skin, or by the anti-inflammatory effect of antibiotics. Increased levels of CD1a and cathelicidin LL-37 may have a critical role in rosacea pathogenesis.

## 3.2. Common Side Effects and Adverse Reactions

This has been reviewed by two subsequent Cochrane reviews, which concluded that long-term treatment of rosacea patients using topical or systemic antibiotics could result in control of the severity of the condition. In trials of the treatment of mild-to-moderate papulopustular rosacea, recruitment bias was noted: enrolled patients were untypical of those seen in clinical practice in retaining an interest in using antibiotics, or that the patients were unhappy with previous activity due to infections - and such studies were often too short to assess the development of antibiotic resistance. It is important when developing effective treatment strategies to consider the common side effects and any adverse reactions which may occur in patients, in addition to the risk of resistance.

Antibiotics have long been a mainstay in the treatment of rosacea. Physicians frequently use them to treat inflammatory lesions and ocular rosacea, while some advocate their use for erythrotelangiectatic rosacea given the common features between these two wider sub-phenotypes. These are generally well-tolerated, with common side effects such as gastrointestinal problems, including diarrhea or upset stomach. There are also reports of opportunistic infections, yeast infections, and allergic reactions. As antibiotics are typically given over long periods of time to treat rosacea, the Society and AAD guidelines routinely call for blood tests to exclude other conditions, such as lupus or liver disease, especially when using drugs which may lead to these side effects.

## 4. Combination Therapy: Antibiotics and Lifestyle Changes

One feature should be noted here: bioactive substances which play a role in immune function are of potential value in disease condition, not only in their deficient form but also in their overdose. It is the same with the role of antibiotics. A combination of several stress-reduction techniques may provide the best answer for a patient with rosacea. Stress reduction plays a major role in improving rosacea. The combination of multiple stress management techniques (e.g., pharmaceutical, skin care, and anti-inflammatory products) will be the keystones. It will be necessary to work with families and children in the household to provide a more effective intervention program, with psychological and nervous support for family rosacea members. The goal is to minimize CO and CO, and ultimately, in defining the treatment process, to enhance the quality of life.

Using two or more treatment modalities harmoniously to treat the same illness condition can, in pharmacological sense, be considered as a way of synergism. It has been proposed that multiple factors contribute to the etiology of rosacea. The idea of employing antibiotic therapy in combination with lifestyle changes seems to be right in line with the concept of treating the syndrome of rosacea. Diet, nutrition, and dietary supplements such as omega-3 fatty acids have also been addressed as potential courses to follow rosacea.

## 4.1. Impact of Diet and Nutrition on Rosacea Symptoms

A focus on diet may be important in the treatment of rosacea patients, as diet triggers are associated with specific gut metabolites. The diet significantly affects gut microbiota and its metabolites. A Western diet may increase inflammation and insulin resistance in acne. Dietary changes may cause alterations in glucose metabolism. Other systemic effects of diet, such as increased gut leakiness and increased stress, may influence the gut-brain-skin connections. The aim of treating patients is to decrease the symptoms, the effects of these substances, and the systemic effects of these substances.

In addition to antibiotics, several other lifestyle factors also affect the symptoms of rosacea, such as severe flushing, persistent redness, bumps and pimples, visible blood vessels, and irritation. Although not all individuals with rosacea may have the same triggers, there are a number of foods that have been commonly associated with causing flare-ups among those with rosacea. There are many websites with lists of foods and recipes for individuals with rosacea that claim to be safe. There are also surveys and research studies that note that many people with rosacea avoid spices, alcohol, and hot drinks. While there continue to be debates in the medical community about diet and nutrition in rosacea and antibiotic effects, many still believe that rosacea should be treated with a more unified approach. The influence of antibiotics cannot be studied independently of other factors, since various environmental factors can adversely influence the gut microbiota.

## 4.2. Stress Management Techniques and Their Role in Treatment

One way to further elucidate the ad hoc hypothesis that stress management techniques may sometimes be an important part of treatment for rosacea would be to conduct a study where we give one population of participants with rosacea doxycycline, and give another population the same antibiotic medication in addition to some form of stress management that had not yet been tried. Then, one would compare the results of these two populations of participants to see whether implementing the specifics of a stress management technique shows significant improvement. A study of that kind would be a good first step. What kind of stress management technique or treatments could be employed in such studies? As detailed by the National Rosacea Society expert committee and as supported by a survey of the published data on the subject, available therapeutic agents could be generally branched into four categories: "cognitive techniques such as meditation," "behavioral techniques such as biofeedback and relaxation," "physical or somatic techniques such as massage or yoga," and "social techniques...[which] promote the value of social support and wellness in the healing process." The same survey found that both of the control groups that were currently investigated in double-blind trials have also been determined to be effective: written intervention using behavioral techniques and videos on rosacea.

Given that some authors now propose that rosaceans be treated with both antibiotics and other therapies to manage what is increasingly seen as a comprehensive symptom complex, it is relevant to consider how much benefit might be obtained from stress management techniques when such techniques are used as an adjunct to or in combination with antibiotics. This section will explore the present data found in the literature on the effectiveness of such techniques in treating a diverse array of so-called "rosacea" symptoms that are sometimes present in those with pustular or ocular rosacea.

# 5. Future Directions and Emerging Therapies

Probiotic interventions - consumption of live microorganisms has been shown to improve clinical outcomes in a wide range of immune, gastrointestinal, and dermatological conditions. While rosacea has become an illness partly characterized by an altered microbiome cutis, intervention with beneficial microorganisms, i.e., "probiotics," is as yet an experimental treatment. Only a few meager scientific reports on humans existing to date, different from ter, show some signs of probiotic treatment as being effective, but more evidence is needed to hammer out this therapeutic approach. New, controlled clinical trials are needed to estimate the cost-effective management of rosacea. Furthermore, it is important to determine the extent and nature of dietary influence on rosacea.

Novel antibiotic formulations - reviewing currently available antibiotics is important because of growing concerns of bacterial resistance, and the side effects associated with oral tetracyclines are of clinical relevance. Microsurgical injectable devices could provide improved outcomes due to more precise application, even antibiotic biodistribution, potency, and pharmacologic effects as the lower amount of antibiotic can be used in therapy. A novel device (Xydalba) has been developed to directly release antibiotics in dermal and subdermal tissues. Retapamulin i.i, a mouse-focused bactericidal treatment option, requires new conductance and could potentially offer new properties in rosacea treatment. Future studies should evaluate the efficacy and safety of these new treatment regimens.

Future directions and emerging therapies in rosacea management

## 5.1. Novel Antibiotic Formulations and Delivery Systems

In areas outside of dermatology, intensifying the "classical" antibiotic activity of a product can be achieved in various ways. Clinically speaking, combination therapy appears to be a more promising approach as the respective action of the two drugs could provide symptomatic relief from the inflammation and erythema associated with rosacea. The non-antibiotic antimicrobial properties of retrocycline can decrease the severity of papules and pustules in rosacea patients. The combination of anti-inflammatory and anti-acne agents in a single formulation product presents appealing advantages. Topical arsenical medications have been largely proven to be anti-inflammatory drugs and the formulation of sodium thioarsenate with salicylic acid has been marketed for decades to address various skin irritation and inflammation problems, such as pityriasis lichenoides and acne.

Rosacea has a considerable impact on a patient's quality of life, owing to its chronic and recurrent nature, its varied and often uncontrolled manifestations, and its independent association with depression, anxiety, and other psychiatric disturbances. Topical and oral antibiotics represent historical cornerstones of rosacea management. In the last decade, many scientific contributions have assessed the inflammatory and non-antibiotic effects of macrolides, tetracyclines, and related compounds: this knowledge has inspired some drug-makers. The search for innovative tactics which are able to boost the efficacy of specific antibiotic formulations and reduce the likelihood of severe side effects has gained significant traction. The purpose of this section is to critically review the recent literature on novel antibiotic formulations, antimicrobials with a non-antibiotic MOA, and technological solutions for enhancing antibiotic skin penetration in patients with rosacea.

## 5.2. Exploring the Potential of Probiotics in Rosacea Management

When deeply looking at probiotic possibilities, there is also a truly novel speculation that reveals a potential to apply an expanded array of treatments in rosacea management. Potential of microbial cross-talk in rosacea conditions with the hypothesis is supported by the known act of the antibiotic minocycline, which suppresses papule formation by reducing the vascular endothelial growth factor (VEGF) expression in skin. As mentioned earlier, such a potential has already been partially proven in the case of neurodermatitis, which is similar to rosacea in terms of its probable pathogenesis, with a decrease in SCORAD, a reduced expression of S. aureus in the skin, and lower levels of the pro-inflammatory IL-6 and COX-2 post-treatment. If the development of such a treatment in rosacea patients is corroborated, it could expand the preventative and therapeutic activity offered.

Despite the countless studies highlighting the role of oral and topical antibiotics in managing the key symptoms of rosacea, with dose-finding studies illustrating minimum effective concentrations of tetracyclines, the search for alternative therapeutic interventions in the management of rosacea symptoms is ongoing. To acknowledge all the aforementioned points, this review is aimed at focusing on scientific evidence and case reports that explore the potential of an alternative treatment – probiotics. It is hypothesized that the chosen direction will allow us to see a new gateway opening to safer and simultaneously holistic approaches in the management of rosacea. Although there are obstacles in the way of corroborating our hypothesis, there is undoubtedly some novel evidence supporting the therapeutic possibility of using a completely new direction in the management of rosacea patients. It was therefore decided to prepare a review comparing the use of probiotics and antibiotics in rosacea treatment.